Calendar 2025

January

MO	TU	WE	TH	FR	SA	SU
		1	2	3	4	5
6	7	8	9	10	11	12
13	14	15	16	17	18	19
20	21	22	23	24	25	26
27	28	29	30	31		

Fabruary

MO	TU	WE	TH	FR	SA	SU
					1	2
3	4	5	6	7	8	9
10	11	12	13	14	15	16
17	18	19	20	21	22	23
24	25	26	27	28		

March

MO	TU	WE	TH	FR	SA	SU
					1	2
3	4	5	6	7	8	9
10	11	12	13	14	15	16
17	18	19	20	21	22	23
24	25	26	27	28	29	30
31						

April

MO	TU	WE	TH	FR	SA	SU
	1	2	3	4	5	6
7	8	9	10	11	12	13
14	15	16	17	18	19	20
21	22	23	24	25	26	27
28	29	30				

May

MO	TU	WE	TH	FR	SA	SU
			1	2	3	4
5	6	7	8	9	10	11
12	13	14	15	16	17	18
19	20	21	22	23	24	25
26	27	28	29	30	31	

June

MO	TU	WE	TH	FR	SA	SU
						1
2	3	4	5	6	7	8
9	10	11	12	13	14	15
16	17	18	19	20	21	22
23	24	25	26	27	28	29
30						

July

MO	TU	WE	TH	FR	SA	SU
	1	2	3	4	5	6
7	8	9	10	11	12	13
14	15	16	17	18	19	20
21	22	23	24	25	26	27
28	29	30	31			

August

MO	TU	WE	TH	FR	SA	SU
				1	2	3
4	5	6	7	8	9	10
11	12	13	14	15	16	17
18	19	20	21	22	23	24
25	26	27	28	29	30	31

September

MO	TU	WE	TH	FR	SA	SU
1	2	3	4	5	6	7
8	9	10	11	12	13	14
15	16	17	18	19	20	21
22	23	24	25	26	27	28
29	30					

October

MO	TU	WE	TH	FR	SA	SU
	1	2	3	4	5	
6	7	8	9	10	11	12
13	14	15	16	17	18	19
20	21	22	23	24	25	26
27	28	29	30	31		

November

MO	TU	WE	TH	FR	SA	SU
					1	2
3	4	5	6	7	8	9
10	11	12	13	14	15	16
17	18	19	20	21	22	23
24	25	26	27	28	29	30

December

MO	TU	WE	TH	FR	SA	SU
1	2	3	4	5	6	7
8	9	10	11	12	13	14
15	16	17	18	19	20	21
22	23	24	25	26	27	28
29	30	31				

All About Me

MY FULL NAME IS

I LIKE TO BE CALLED

MY BIRTHDAY IS

I LIVE WITH MY

FOR FUN, I LIKE TO

MY FRIENDS' NAMES ARE

THIS YEAR, I HOPE TO LEARN ABOUT

WHEN I GROW UP, I WANT TO BE

HOW TO SELF-CARE

Get creative

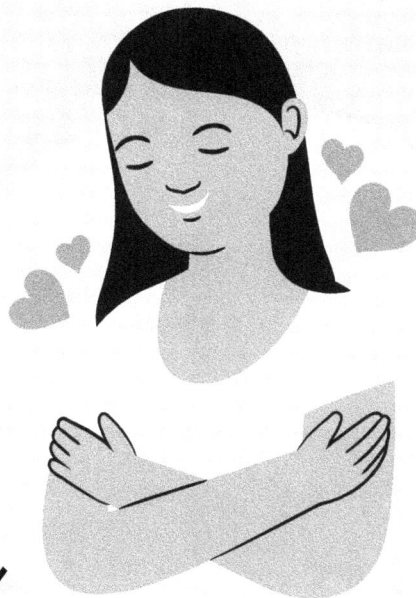

Social media detox

Listen to music

Face mask & skincare routine

Bubble bath

MENTAL HEALTH

Tips For Taking Care Of Your

Talk To Someone You Trust

Take Care Of Your Physical Health

Do Activities That You Enjoy

Take Two Minutes To Focus On The World Around You

Don't Be Afraid To Say "No"

Tell Yourself That Everything Will Be Fine

MENTAL HEALTH

Tips For Taking Care Of You

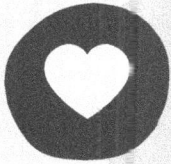

- Talk To Someone You Trust

- Take Care Of Your Physical Health

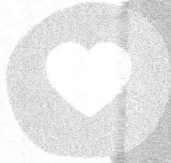

- Do Activities That You Enjoy

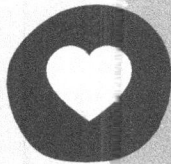

- Take Two Minutes To Focus On The World Around You

- Tell Yourself That Everything Will Be Fine

3 TIPS FOR A HAPPY LIFE

1. ## Be Grateful Every Day

   Reflecting on positive things and writing in a gratitude journal can increase happiness and satisfaction.

2. ## Maintain Good Social Relations

   Spending time with family and friends provides emotional support and increases feelings of happiness.

3. ## Do Activities You Enjoy

   Doing hobbies and activities you love gives you a sense of accomplishment and satisfaction.

Mental Health Tips

FOR BUSINESS LEADERS

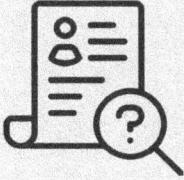

BECOME A PROFICIENT OBSERVER

1

It's easy to justify our feelings by telling ourselves, but the real trick is challenging those thoughts.

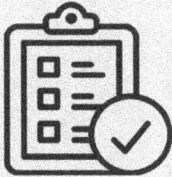

TAKE ACTION BEFORE YOU HIT ROCK BOTTOM

2

Whenever you notice you're slipping, this is the time to do something about it.

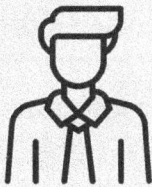

LEAD BY EXAMPLE FOR YOUR STAFF

3

It can empower your colleagues when you look after your own mental health.

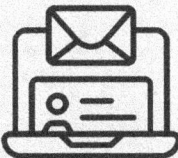

KNOWING THE SERVICES AVAILABLE

4

There is a lot of online support for mental health, making it easier to talk and gain confidence.

These 4 tips
Will Help You Manage
Your Mental Health

Plan daily mental health activities

Remember to refuel your brain and body with nutrition to keep them functioning.

Being prepared and planning your time helps you avoid being overwhelmed.

Feel free to express yourself

Manage stress proactively

The release of uncom fortable emotions can help you manage maintain mental health.

Humans are hardwired to desire meaningful connections with others.

Friendly with others

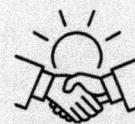

TIPS FOR MAINTAINING
MENTAL HEALTH

DON'T GIVE
UP ON YOUR
DREAM

DON'T BE
AFRAID TO
SAY "NO"

CONNECT WITH
OTHERS AND BE
SOCIABLE

DON'T BE
TO HARD ON
YOURSELF

BELIEVE
YOURSELF

ASK
FOR
HELP

5 Ways To Be MINDFUL

1 Focus on what is happening around you. What do you see, hear, smell, taste, or feel?

2 Take deep breaths and count each time you breathe in and breathe out.

3 Show yourself some compassion by thinking kind thoughts about yourself.

4 Think of a person or place that makes you happy. What brings you joy?

5 Find a quiet activity that makes you feel calm and allows you to focus your attention.

5 Ways of Thinking
That Will Improve Your Life

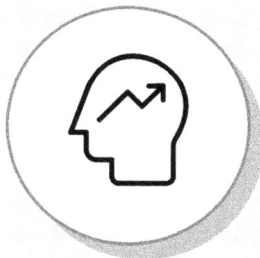

01

A Growth Mindset

Believe that you can grow and develop with effort, practice, and learning.

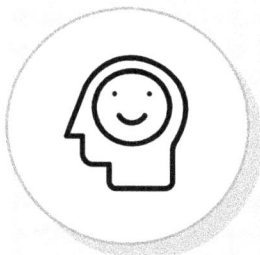

02

A Positive Mindset

Focus on the good things in your life and work to turn negative thinking into positive thinking.

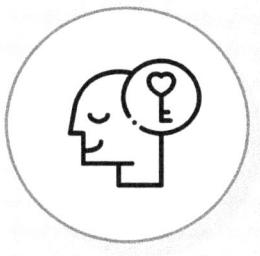

03

An Open Mindset

Strive to remain open-minded by considering different perspectives and challenging your own beliefs.

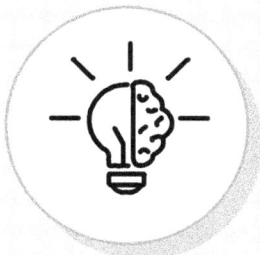

04

A Creative Mindset

Looking at problems from a different perspective can often lead to innovative solutions.

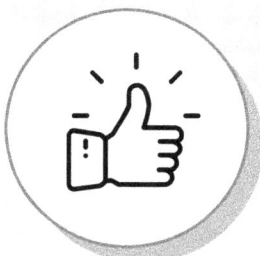

05

A Confident Mindset

Developing a confident mindset will help you take on challenges with courage and enthusiasm.

5 Minute Gratitude Journal

S M T W T H F S

Breath before writing

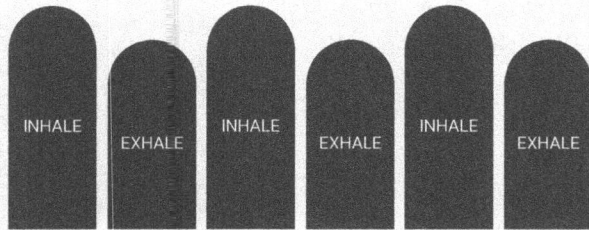

INHALE EXHALE INHALE EXHALE INHALE EXHALE

3 best thing about today

Things you're grateful today

- ☐ _____
- ☐ _____
- ☐ _____
- ☐ _____
- ☐ _____

Describe today in a drawing

Today's Highlight

Things that you learned

Today's Affirmation

_____

_____

DAILY HEALTH

DATE:_ _ _ / _ _ _ /_ _ _ _

BODY CARE: _____

BREAKFAST	
LUNCH	
DINNER	

SNACK

SPORT
♥
◉
🔋
🥛

DON'T FORGET

1 _____

2 _____

3 _____

SLEEP AT	WAKE UP AT

MENTAL CARE: _____

TODAY WAS	TOMORROW WILL

APPOINTMENTS

VISION BOARD

Career

Finance

Relationships

Love

Personal Growth

Health

Leisure

Home

Self-Care
Planner

DATE _____ / _____ / _____

S	M	T	W	T	F	S

TODAY'S ACTIVITIES

- _____
- _____
- _____
- _____
- _____
- _____
- _____
- _____
- _____
- _____
- _____
- _____

WEATHER :

MOOD :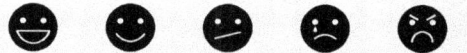

WATER BALANCE :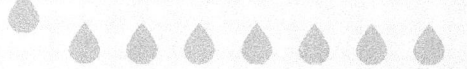

Things that make me happy today
_____

HOURS OF SLEEP

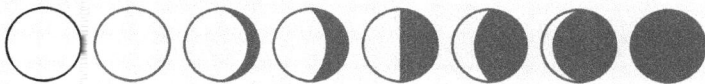

SLEEPLESS ————→ FULLY CHARGED

GOALS FOR TOMORROW

MY SELF-CARE CHECKLIST

TASKS	SU	MO	TU	WE	TH	FR	SA
Wake up at 8am	✓	○	○	○	○	○	○
Drink water 8 glasses	○	○	○	○	○	○	○
Do yoga	○	○	○	○	○	○	○
Get some fresh air	○	○	○	○	○	○	○
Eat healthy breakfast	○	○	○	○	○	○	○
Make a plan for the day	○	○	○	○	○	○	○
Take a hot shower	○	○	○	○	○	○	○
Walking 30 minutes	○	○	○	○	○	○	○
Workout 30 minutes	○	○	○	○	○	○	○
Play some music	○	○	○	○	○	○	○
Read a book	○	○	○	○	○	○	○
Smile and laugh	○	○	○	○	○	○	○
Unplug for a while	○	○	○	○	○	○	○
Get a good night sleep	○	○	○	○	○	○	○

Daily
Gratitude

Things you are grateful for today

_____

_____

_____

_____

_____

MORE OF THIS:

Affirmations

- _____
- _____
- _____
- _____
- _____

LESS OF THIS:

GRATITUDE

MONTHLY
PREVIEW   DATE ___ /___ /___

THIS MONTH'S INTENTION IS

_____

_____

_____

HOW DO YOU FEEL?

_____

_____

_____

_____

_____

_____

HOW DO YOU WANT TO FEEL?

_____

_____

_____

_____

_____

WHERE DO YOU WANT TO FOCUS YOUR ENERGY?

_____

_____

Notes:

_____

_____

GRATITUDE
MONTHLY
REVIEW: DATE ___ /___ /___

HIGHLIGHTS OF THE MONTH

1 _____

2 _____

3 _____

WHAT IS SOMETHING NEW YOU'VE LEARNED?

_____

_____

_____

WHAT WERE SOME OF THE CHALLENGES YOU FACED?

_____

_____

_____

WHAT IS THE BEST THING YOU HAVE DONE FOR YOURSELF THIS PAST MONTH?

_____

_____

_____

HAS PRACTICING GRATITUDE HELPED YOU THIS MONTH?

| YES | MAYBE | NO |

DAILY PLANNER

M	T	W	T	F	S	S

TIME	ACTIVITY
06:00	
07:00	
08:00	
09:00	
10:00	
11:00	
12:00	
13:00	
14:00	
15:00	
16:00	
17:00	
18:00	
19:00	
20:00	

3 MAIN TASKS

TO DO LIST

REMARK

WEEKLY PLANNER

DATE: _____

MONDAY: _____

_____

_____

_____

TUESDAY: _____

_____

_____

_____

WEDNESDAY: _____

_____

_____

_____

THURSDAY: _____

_____

_____

_____

FRIDAY: _____

_____

_____

_____

SATURDAY: _____

_____

_____

_____

WEEKEND

_____

_____

_____

_____

_____

TO-DO LISTS

_____

_____

_____

_____

_____

_____

NOTE

_____

_____

_____

_____

_____

_____

_____

_____

_____

Monthly Planner

Month: _____   Year: _____

Mon	Tue	Wed	Thu	Fri	Sat	Sun

Top Priorities

_____

_____

Notes

_____

_____

Self-Care
CHECKLIST

DATE ___ / ___ / ___

S	M	T	W	T	F	S

- ◯ HEALTHY MEALS
- ◯ GO FOR A WALK
- ◯ CLEANING HOUSE
- ◯ WASHING CLOTHES
- ◯ LISTEN TO MUSIC
- ◯ HAVE A POWER NAP
- ◯ MAKE YOUR BED
- ◯ TAKE YOUR MEDICATIONS & VITAMINS
- ◯ SKINCARE ROUTINE
- ◯ SOCIAL MEDIA BREAK
- ◯ TAKE A LONG BATH
- ◯ DO A FACE MASK
- ◯ CALL A FRIEND OR FAMILY
- ◯ MEDITATION
- ◯ WATCH A MOVIE
- ◯ CUDDLE A PET OR HUMAN
- ◯ TRY A NEW RESTAURANT
- ◯ MAKE TIME TO READ
- ◯ TRY A NEW RECIPE
- ◯ NO PHONE 30 MINS BEFORE BED

WEATHER :

MOOD :

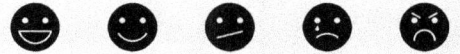

WATER BALANCE :

HOURS OF SLEEP

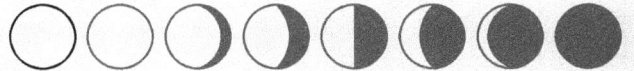

*Things that make
me happy today*

Self-Care Practice

Name :

Date :

Physical Self-care

EMOTIONAL SELF-CARE

SPIRITUAL SELF-CARE

Things I like

Intellectual Self-care

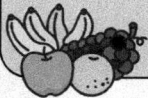

Things I don't like

Social Self-care

Financial Self-care

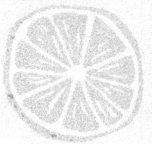

30 DAY
SELF CARE CHALLENGE

MONTH:

YEAR:

take a 10 minute walk outside

practice deep breathing for 5 minutes

drink a glass of water

learn yoga for beginner

listen to your favorite song

stretch for 5 minutes

have a healthy snack

meditate for 10 minutes

call a friend or family member

take a power nap

do a quick decluttering session

watch a funny video

read a few pages of a book

do a quick workout

have a soothing cup of tea

try a new recipe

write in a journal for 5 minutes

do a random act of kindness

take a relaxing bath

unplug from technology for an hour

watch the sunset or sunrise

do a mini DIY project

make some word of affirmation

dance to your favorite music

reflect on your day before going to bed

notes

goals

SELF CARE INTENTION

MONTH:

YEAR:

PHYSICAL SELF CARE

EMOTION SELF CARE

SPIRITUAL SELF CARE

SOCIAL SELF CARE

NOTE TO SELF

Self-Care Assessment

SPIRITUAL SELF-CARE

1	2	3	★	Pray
				Meditate
				Spend time in nature
				Act in accordance with my morals and values
				Participate in a cause that is important to me

1	2	3	★	Profesional Self-Care
				Take breaks during work
				Improve my professional skills
				Overal professional self-care
				Adviocate for fair pay, benefits, and other needs
				Take on project that are interesting or rewarding

Self Reflection Questions

What are my goals in my life?

_____

What are my strengths?

_____

What do i love about my self?

_____

Who matters the most to me?

_____

What am i ashamed of?

_____

What do i like to do for fun?

_____

What am i worried about?

_____

Where do i feel safest?

_____

Who gives me comfort?

_____

What is my happiest memory?

_____

What keeps my grounded?

_____

What am i grateful for?

_____

Health Habit

	MENU PLANNER	WORKOUT	WATER INTAKE
MONDAY	Breakfast Lunch Dinner Snacks	Exercise Calories Burned	
TUESDAY	Breakfast Lunch Dinner Snacks	Exercise Calories Burned	
WEDNESDAY	Breakfast Lunch Dinner Snacks	Exercise Calories Burned	
THURSDAY	Breakfast Lunch Dinner Snacks	Exercise Calories Burned	
FRIDAY	Breakfast Lunch Dinner Snacks	Exercise Calories Burned	
SATURDAY	Breakfast Lunch Dinner Snacks	Exercise Calories Burned	
SUNDAY	Breakfast Lunch Dinner Snacks	Exercise Calories Burned	

Self-Care Challenge Checklist

	M	T	W	T	F	S	S
Meditate for 10 min							
Deep breathing							
Walk for at least 15 min							
Talk to friends							
Journal for 15 min							
Listen to a podcast or read a book							
Exercise or run for 30 min							
Healthy diet							
Take vitamins							
No technology 30 min before bedtime							
7-8 hours of sleep							

NOTES

_____

_____

Self-Care Tracker

DATE ___ /___ /___

Morning Rituals	S	M	T	W	T	F	S

Night Rituals	S	M	T	W	T	F	S

Sleep Tracker

DATE	6	7	8	9	10	11	12	1	2	3	4	5	6	7	8	9	10	11	12

Habit Tracker

HABITS

	M	T	W	T	F	S	S
	☐	☐	☐	☐	☐	☐	☐
	☐	☐	☐	☐	☐	☐	☐
	☐	☐	☐	☐	☐	☐	☐
	☐	☐	☐	☐	☐	☐	☐
	☐	☐	☐	☐	☐	☐	☐
	☐	☐	☐	☐	☐	☐	☐
	☐	☐	☐	☐	☐	☐	☐
	☐	☐	☐	☐	☐	☐	☐
	☐	☐	☐	☐	☐	☐	☐
	☐	☐	☐	☐	☐	☐	☐

Goals

Daily Wellness Log

Daily Affirmation

Water Tracker

Exercise Log

Mood Tracker

Meals

Breakfast

Lunch

Dinner

Snacks

Drinks

Daily Affirmation

Today I am grateful for

1.

2.

3.

Things I can do to make today great

1.

2.

3.

Great things that happened today

1.

2.

3.

Thoughts and Reflections

Daily Self-love Journal

Mood: ☹ 🙁 😐 🙂 😃   DATE: ___ /___ /___

EMPOWERING
AFFIRMATION

TODAY, I FORGIVE MYSELF FOR...

I FEEL GOOD ABOUT MYSELF
BECAUSE...

REMINDER

REFLECTION

_____

_____

_____

_____

_____

_____

_____

_____

Weekly self love journal

Mood: 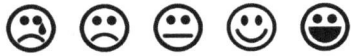   DATE ___ / ___ / ___

Monday

Three positive things about me...

Tuesday

I feel good about myself when...

Wednesday

Things I should do when I'm sad...

Thursday

Things I should do when I'm Bored...

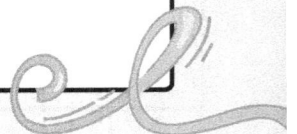

Weekly self love journal

Mood: 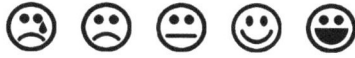 DATE ____ /____ /____

Friday

Things I should do when I feel tired...

Saturday

Things that made me happy today...

Sunday

I will challenge myself to...

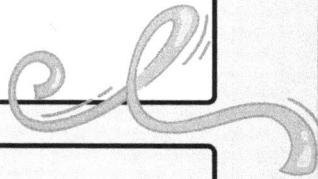

Notes:

Brain Dump

MONTH:

TOPIC	

THOUGHTS

_____
_____
_____
_____
_____
_____
_____

IDEAS

ACTION STEPS

- [ ] _____
- [ ] _____
- [ ] _____
- [ ] _____
- [ ] _____
- [ ] _____
- [ ] _____
- [ ] _____
- [ ] _____
- [ ] _____
- [ ]

Goal Tracker 🎯

Goal 1:

Start Date
_____

End Date
_____

My Why
_____

_____

_____

Action Steps
○ _____
○ _____
○ _____
○ _____

Notes
_____
_____
_____
_____

Goal 2:

Start Date
_____

End Date
_____

My Why
_____

_____

_____

Action Steps
○ _____
○ _____
○ _____
○ _____

Notes
_____
_____
_____
_____

Goal 3:

Start Date
_____

End Date
_____

My Why
_____

_____

_____

Action Steps
○ _____
○ _____
○ _____
○ _____

Notes
_____
_____
_____
_____

Goal 4:

Start Date
_____

End Date
_____

My Why
_____

_____

_____

Action Steps
○ _____
○ _____
○ _____
○ _____

Notes
_____
_____
_____
_____

Medication Tracker

Date	Medication	Dose	Frequency	Time

MEDICAL HISTORY

Name :
Age :
Blood Group :
Primary Doctor :
Allergies :
Chronic Conditions :

DATE	ILLNESS / SURGERIES	DOCTOR / HOSPITAL

Doctor Visits

DATE ____ / ____ / ____

Time : 🕐

PATIENT :

HOSPITAL :

DOCTOR :

CONTACT INFO :

LOCATION :

AGE :

HEIGHT :

WEIGHT :

HEART RATE :

BLOOD PRESSURE :

REASON FOR VISIT

DOCTOR'S COMMENTS

PRESCRIPTION & INSTRUCTIONS

Medical Condition

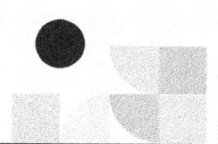

PATIENT		DOCTOR	
AGE / GENDER		TEMPERATURE	
WEIGHT		HEART RATE	
HEIGHT		BLOOD PREASURE	

DATE	TREATMENT	DESCRIPTION

MEDICAL NOTE

ALLERGIES

Medical Appointment

DATE		TIME	
DOCTOR		SPECIALITY	
ADDRESS			
REASON FOR VISIT			

DATE		TIME	
DOCTOR		SPECIALITY	
ADDRESS			
REASON FOR VISIT			

DATE		TIME	
DOCTOR		SPECIALITY	
ADDRESS			
REASON FOR VISIT			

DATE		TIME	
DOCTOR		SPECIALITY	
ADDRESS			
REASON FOR VISIT			

EMERGENCY HOSPITAL VISIT

Arrival		TIME:

DATE:_ _ /_ _ _ /_ _ _

NAME:

DOCTOR:

DEPARTMENT:

ASSISTANT:

CASE

TESTS & RESULTS

MEDICATION ISSUED

NOTES

FIRST AID INFOSHEET

First Aid Kit Location:

Inventory List	Qty

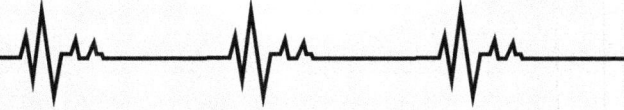

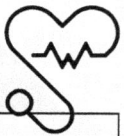

Burn injury first aid :

Seizure first aid :

Stroke first aid :

Heart attack first aid :

Period Tracker

	J	F	M	A	M	J	J	A	S	O	N	D
1												
2												
3												
4												
5												
6												
7												
8												
9												
10												
11												
12												
13												
14												
15												
16												
17												
18												
19												
20												
21												
22												
23												
24												
25												
26												
27												
28												
29												
30												
31												

SYMPTOMS KEY

- ☐ Spotting
- ☐ Light
- ☐ Medium
- ☐ Heavy
- ☐ Acne
- ☐ Cramps
- ☐ Cravings
- ☐ Fatigue
- ☐ Headache

Things to Avoid

NOTE

ANXIETY BREAKDOWN

Name:	Date:

What is making you feel anxious?

What thoughts are going through your head?

How is your body responding?

What is the worst thing that can happen?

In this case, what is under your control?

What can you do to calm your body?

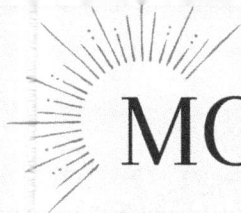

MORNING ROUTINE

- [ ] *no phone for the first 30 min*
- [ ] *journal 3 things you are grateful for*
- [ ] *make the bed*
- [ ] *drink a glass of water*
- [ ] *10 minutes stretch*
- [ ] *short meditation*
- [ ] *shower (or cold shower)*
- [ ] *take vitamins/food supplements*
- [ ] *make breakfast and coffee*
- [ ] *read a book or magazine*
- [ ] *review your schedule for the day*
- [ ] *write down a to-do list*
- [ ] *enjoy your day!*

My Bedtime Routine

(Tick off after you finished the routine)

- ☐ CLEAN UP THE WORKSPACE

- ☐ BRUSH TEETH & WASH FACE

- ☐ APPLY SKINCARE ROUTINE

- ☐ CHANGE UP TO PAJAMA

- ☐ WRITE TO-DO LIST FOR TOMORROW

- ☐ DRINK WARM WATER

- ☐ JOURNALING

- ☐ TAKE A QUICK MEDITATION

SELF-REFLECTION JOURNAL

DATE:_ _ /_ _ _ /_ _ _

MONTH:

How am I feeling today?

Great   Good   Okay   Not Good

★ THINGS TO BE DONE FOR TODAY ★

★ Today, I'm grateful for

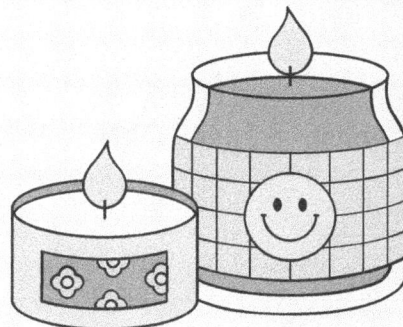

Today's water intake | 1 | 2 | 3 | 4 | 5 | 6 | 7 |

★ Best Things Happened Today

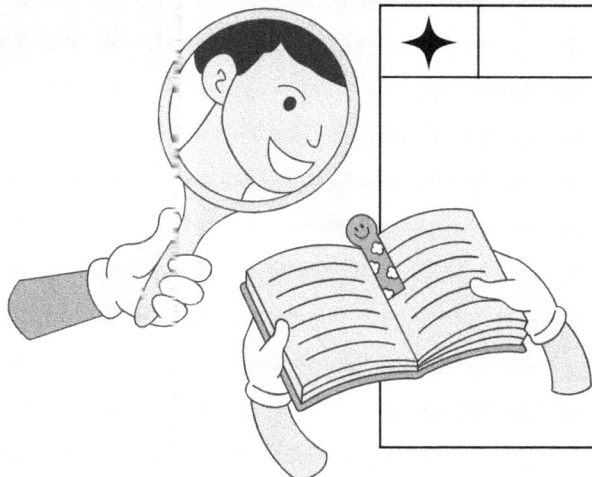

VISION BOARD

CAREER

FINANCE

RELATIONSHIPS

LOVE

PERSONAL GROWTH

HEALTH

LEISURE

HOME

VISION BOARD

WEALTH:

1.
2.
3.
4.
5.
6.
7.
8.
9.
10.

HEALTH:

1.
2.
3.
4.
5.
6.
7.
8.
9.
10.

LOVE:

1.
2.
3.
4.
5.
6.
7.
8.
9.
10.

CAREER:

1.
2.
3.
4.
5.
6.
7.
8.
9.
10.

SPIRITUALITY:

1.
2.
3.
4.
5.
6.
7.
8.
9.
10.

FAMILY:

1.
2.
3.
4.
5.
6.
7.
8.
9.
10.

KNOWLEDGE:

1.
2.
3.
4.
5.

BREAK DOWN YOUR GOALS!

NAME: _____   DATE: _____

MY (S)(M)(A)(R)(T) GOAL PLANNER

(S) SPECIFIC ➡

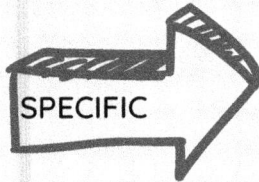

What exactly do I want to accomplish?

(M) MEASURABLE ➡

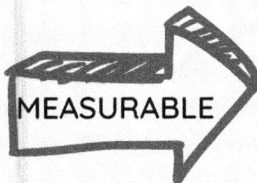

How will I know when I meet my goal?

(A) ATTAINABLE ➡

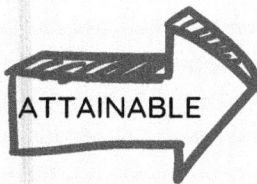

Is it possible to meet this goal with effort by my timeline?

(R) RELEVANT ➡

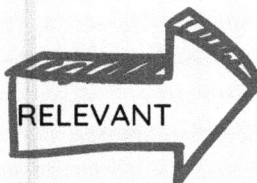

Is this goal worth working hard to accomplish? Does it help me with my long term goals?

(T) TIMELY ➡

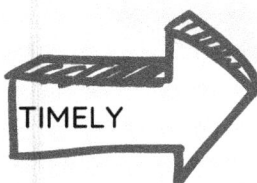

What is the deadline I have set to meet this goal?

MAKE YOUR GOALS SMART
Setting realistic and achievable outcomes.

My goal is:

SPECIFIC

What do I want to happen?

MEASUREABLE

How will I know when I have achieved my goal?

ATTAINABLE

Is the goal realistic and how will I accomplish it?

RELEVANT

Why is my goal important to me?

TIMELY

What is my deadline for this goal?

GOALS PLANNER

Date_____

Goals:

- ● ☐ _____
- ● ☐ _____
- ● ☐ _____
- ● ☐ _____
- ● ☐ _____
- ● ☐ _____
- ● ☐ _____
- ● ☐ _____
- ● ☐ _____
- ● ☐ _____
- ● ☐ _____
- ● ☐ _____
- ● ☐ _____
- ● ☐ _____
- ● ☐ _____
- ● ☐ _____
- ● ☐ _____
- ● ☐ _____

Today's Mood

_____
_____
_____

Goal of the day

_____
_____
_____

Water Intake

_____
_____
_____

Notes / Reminder

_____
_____
_____
_____
_____
_____
_____
_____

● To Start   ☑ Ok   → Delay   ⊘ Stuck   ⊠ Cancel

MY STRENGTHS

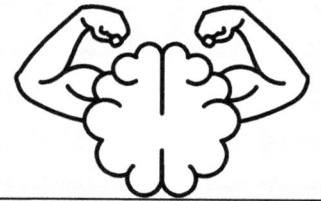

Name:

Things I enjoy doing with my parents

My family make me feel happy and safe when

Things I am good at which. make me happy

I feel most happy about school when

Things my friends do that make me feel happy

In my community, I feel happy and safe when

Self-Care Journal

Date_____

TODAY I'M GRATEFUL FOR:

1. _____

2. _____

3. _____

WATER INTAKE

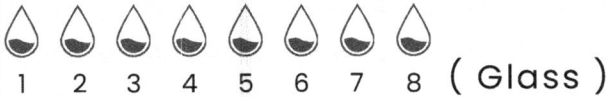

1 2 3 4 5 6 7 8 (Glass)

MOOD

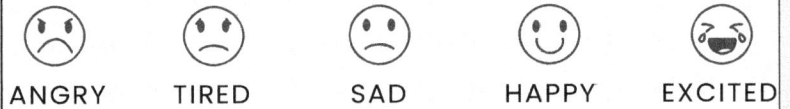

ANGRY   TIRED   SAD   HAPPY   EXCITED

TODAY'S AFFIRMATION

NOTES/REMINDER:

FOR TOMORROW

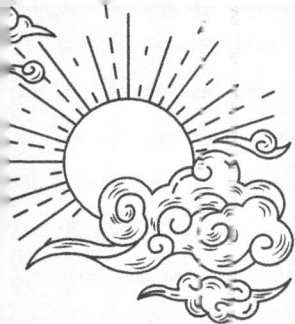

DEAR MY FUTURE SELF

Things to do when I'm sad

Things to do when I'm bored

Today's Date

_____

Dear me,

_____

_____

_____

_____

_____

_____

_____

_____

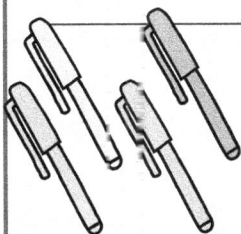

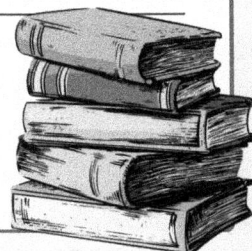

SELF CARE RITUALS

DATE:___ /__ /____

MORNING RITUALS	S	M	T	W	F	S

NIGHT RITUALS	S	M	T	W	F	S

TO DO LIST

MONTH:

DATE:

- [ ]
- [ ]
- [ ]
- [ ]
- [ ]
- [ ]
- [ ]
- [ ]
- [ ]
- [ ]
- [ ]
- [ ]
- [ ]
- [ ]
- [ ]
- [ ]
- [ ]

MY FAVORITE THINGS

We want to learn about your favorite things!
Please fill in the blanks and share your answers with the class.
Don't forget to decorate your worksheet with colors and drawings to make it even more exciting!

My Favorite Color:

_____

My Favorite Animal:

_____

My Favorite Book:

_____

My Favorite hobbie:

_____

My Favorite food:

_____

My Favorite song:

_____

MY FAVORITE PERSON

Who is your favorite person? What is he/she like?
What do you like about him/her? Draw and describe.

MY FAVORITE PLACE

Name: 　　　　　　　　　　　　　　　　　　DATE:___ /__ /____

What's your favorite place to be? Why do you love it?

→

Draw a picture of you in your favorite place.

My Best Vacation Ever

Name:

DATE:___ /__ /____

Draw a special moment and describe your favorite vacation.

GRATITUDE JOURNAL

DATE:_ _ _ / _ _ /_ _ _ _

TODAY I'M GRATEFUL FOR:

TODAY'S AFFIRMATION:

SOMETHING I'M PROUD OF:

WATER INTAKE

NOTES/ REMINDERS

TOMORROW I LOOK FORWARD TO:

My Daily Gratitude Log

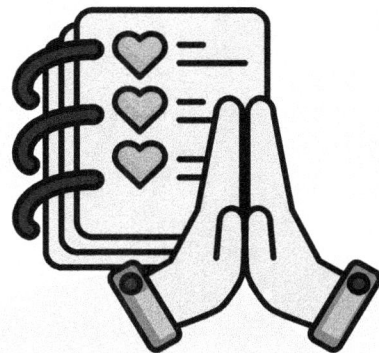

Things you are grateful for today

MORE OF THIS:

LESS OF THIS:

Affirmations

- _____
- _____
- _____
- _____
- _____

30 Days of Gratitude

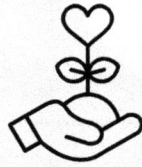

Day 1 _____

Day 2 _____

Day 3 _____

Day 4 _____

Day 5 _____

Day 6 _____

Day 7 _____

Day 8 _____

Day 9 _____

Day 10_____

Day 11_____

Day 12_____

Day 13_____

Day 14_____

Day 15_____

Day 16 _____

Day 17 _____

Day 18 _____

Day 19 _____

Day 20 _____

Day 21 _____

Day 22 _____

Day 23 _____

Day 24 _____

Day 25 _____

Day 26 _____

Day 27 _____

Day 28 _____

Day 29 _____

Day 30 _____

Daily Wellness Log

Daily Affirmation

Water Tracker

Exercise Log

Mood Tracker

Meals

Breakfast

Lunch

Dinner

Snacks

Drinks

Daily Affirmation

Today I am grateful for

1.

2.

3.

Things I can do to make today great

1.

2.

3.

Great things that happened today

1.

2.

3.

Thoughts and Reflections

Daily Gratitude

3 things I'm grateful for today...

1:

2:

3:

What can I learn from today's experiences?

MORNING GRATITUDE

DATE:___ / __ /____

Today I want to feel...

Today I will spread kindness by...

3 things I'm grateful for today are...

"Being happy is a habit."

Evening Gratitude

DATE:_ _ _ / _ _ / _ _ _ _

3 things I'm grateful for today are...

The best part of today was...

What can I learn from today's experiences?

Tomorrow I'm looking forward to...

Mental Health Plan

It matters how you feel about yourself. Put down circumstances and prepare a plan of action for when you'll require assistance.

If...

Then...

If...

Then...

What helps.....

If...

Then...

If...

Then...

What doesn't help.....

MY DAILY MENTAL HEALTH TRACKER

To Do List

-
-
-
-
-

My Mood

- ◯ Sad
- ◯ Happy
- ◯ Angry
- ◯ Afraid

MORNING ROUTINE

-
-
-
-
-

Water Balance

NOTES

Monthly Reflection Journal

DATE:_ _ / _ _ /_ _ _

TIME:

MONTHLY WINS

_____

_____

HOW DOES IT MAKE ME FEEL?

_____

_____

CHALLENGES

_____

_____

HOW CAN I IMPROVE IT?

_____

_____

ACCOMPLISHED GOALS

_____

UNACCOMPLISHED GOALS

_____

GOALS NEXT MONTH

_____

HABITS RETAINED

_____

HABITS ELIMINATED

_____

NEW HABITS DEVELOPED

_____

(GOOD & BAD)

THREE THINGS THAT I AM MOST GRATEFUL FOR THIS MONTH:

Two life lessons I learned this month:

_____

One word that best describes this month:

_____

HOW WILL YOU RATE THIS MONTH? ☆☆☆☆☆

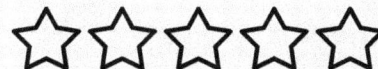

Weekly Cleaning Checklist

	S	M	T	W	T	F	S
Dust furniture	○	○	○	○	○	○	○
Change sheets	○	○	○	○	○	○	○
Clean stovetop	○	○	○	○	○	○	○
Clean mirrors	○	○	○	○	○	○	○
Fold laundry	○	○	○	○	○	○	○
Ironing	○	○	○	○	○	○	○
Empty school bags	○	○	○	○	○	○	○
Mop floors	○	○	○	○	○	○	○
Clean bins	○	○	○	○	○	○	○
Empty fridge	○	○	○	○	○	○	○
Wash blankets	○	○	○	○	○	○	○
Vacuum rugs	○	○	○	○	○	○	○
Clean shower	○	○	○	○	○	○	○
Scrub toilets	○	○	○	○	○	○	○
Clean appliances	○	○	○	○	○	○	○
Declutter living room	○	○	○	○	○	○	○
Clean dining table	○	○	○	○	○	○	○
Wash pet bedding	○	○	○	○	○	○	○
Empty dryer filter	○	○	○	○	○	○	○
Wash towels	○	○	○	○	○	○	○
Mop bathrooms	○	○	○	○	○	○	○
Disinfect sinks	○	○	○	○	○	○	○
Sweep garage	○	○	○	○	○	○	○

Self Love Gratitude

Date:

TODAY'S AFFIRMATION

Today, I am thankful for...

Best part of my day

Quotes

Self Love Planner

TO DO LIST

- ○ _____
- ○ _____
- ○ _____
- ○ _____
- ○ _____
- ○ _____
- ○ _____
- ○ _____

DATE:

Priorities Today

_____

_____

_____

_____

_____

_____

Affirmation

_____

_____

_____

_____

Quotes for Today

_____

_____

_____

_____

PERSONAL REMINDER

_____

_____

_____

_____

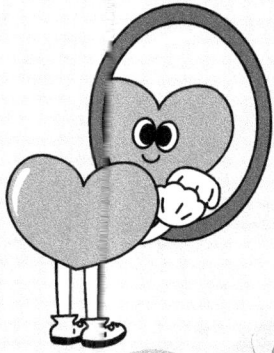

SELF-LOVE
REMINDERS

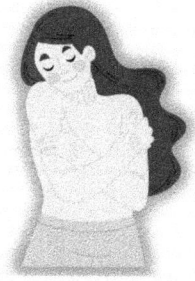

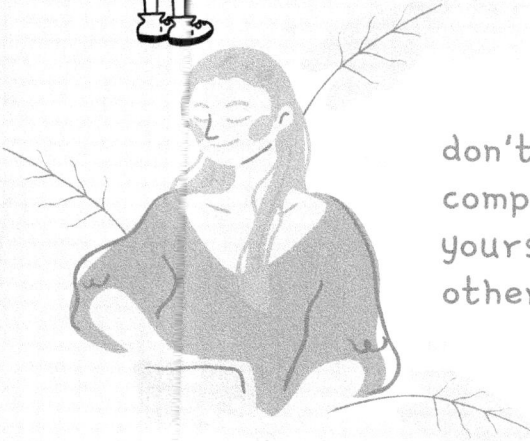

don't compare yourself to others

growing your positive vibe things

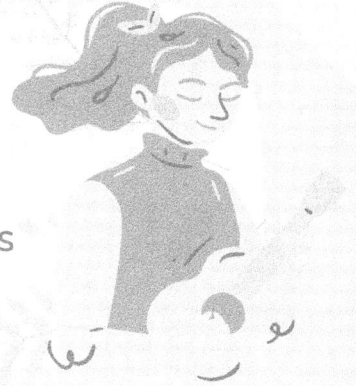

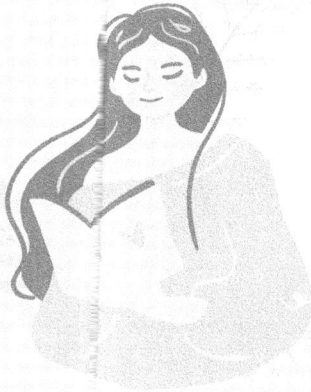

Do an activity you love

Find a place that makes you happy

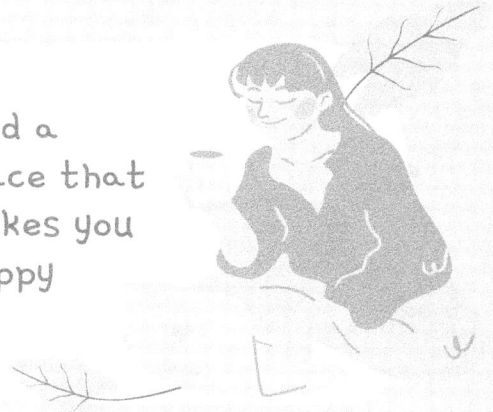

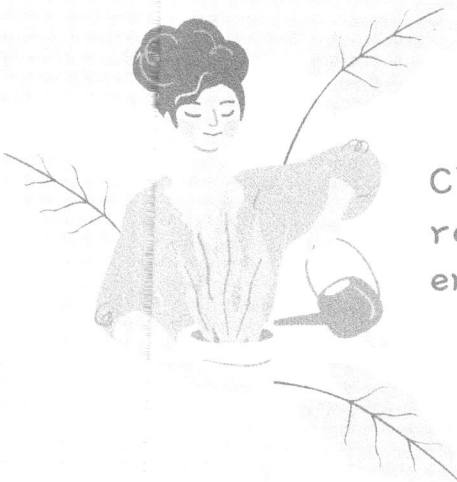

Clean your room and environment

don't forget to take time to relax

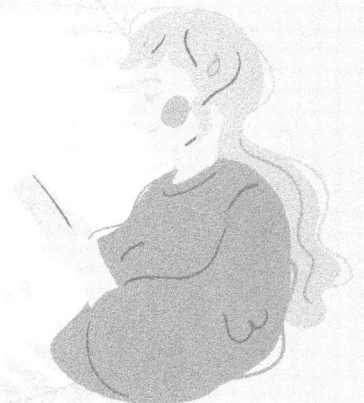

Self Love
Notes

REMINDER

DAILY REFLECTION

Today I am grateful for these three things...
1. A healthy lunch
2. Going to a job that I really enjoy
3. Being able to call a friend who lives so far away

Date: 30 January

Water: 6 glasses

Exercise: 1 hour

Today,
    this good thing happened to me and I appreciate it because:

_____
_____
_____
_____

Today,
    this not so good thing happened to me and this is how I handled it:

_____
_____
_____

Today,
    this thing made me happy:

_____
_____
_____

Today,
    I discovered this about myself:

_____
_____
_____
_____

PERSONAL REFLECTION

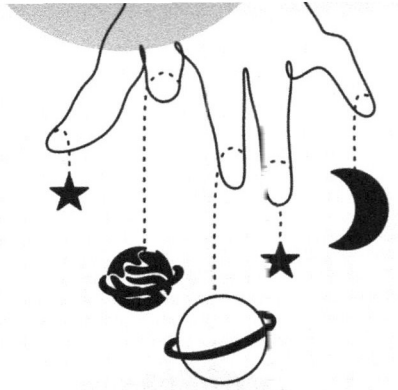

DATE:

THINGS I'M GRATEFUL FOR

BAD HABITS I NEED TO STOP

THINGS THAT MAKE ME FEEL BETTER

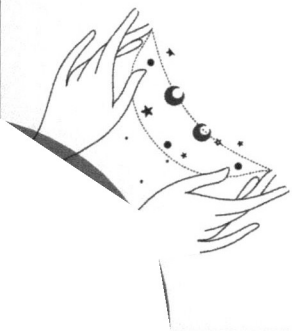

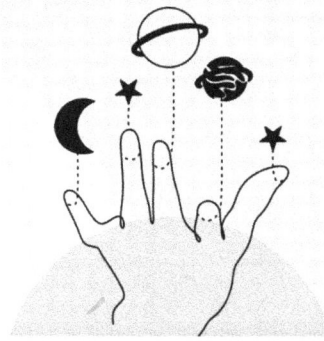

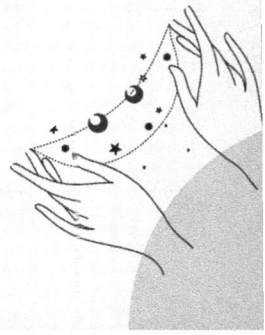

MY SELF EVALUATION

Read each statement below. Place a check mark in the box that best match your behavior in the classroom.

	Always	Sometimes	Never
I follow directions.			
I do my best work.			
I cooperate with others.			
I am polite and respectful to others.			
I complete my work on time.			
I listen to the teacher.			
I raise my hand before I answer questions.			
I participate in class discussions.			
I keep my hands and feet to myself.			

Healthy Weekly Meal Plan

Monday

Tuesday

Wednesday

Thursday

Friday

Saturday

Sunday

Notes

To do List

Goals

Fitness Challenge

Running ⬡ ⬡ ⬡ ⬡ ⬡ ⬡

Strength ⬡ ⬡ ⬡ ⬡ ⬡ ⬡

Yoga ⬡ ⬡ ⬡ ⬡ ⬡ ⬡

Meal Planner

s	Breakfast:	Lunch:	Dinner:
m	Breakfast:	Lunch:	Dinner:
t	Breakfast:	Lunch:	Dinner:
w	Breakfast:	Lunch:	Dinner:
t	Breakfast:	Lunch:	Dinner:
f	Breakfast:	Lunch:	Dinner:
s	Breakfast:	Lunch:	Dinner:

30-DAY HEALTHY EATING CHALLENGE

Chew 30 times	Drink a lot of water	Eat six small meals a day	Eat more fruits	Drink herbal tea
Eat mindfully	Avoid salt	Don't eat processed foods	Laugh and smile	Don't deprive yourself
Take a cold shower	Walk to work	Try a new exercise	Eat more vegetables	Find a supplement
Cook at home	Make homemade food	Grocery shop mindfully	Don't eat past 7 pm	Stretch
Buy a herb plant	Use sunscreen	Take the stairs	Sleep for eight hours	Don't eat refined sugar
Focus on your posture	Give up weighing yourself	Avoid saturated fats	Eat lean meat	Eat whole carbs

WEEKLY MEAL PLAN

s	Breakfast:	Lunch:	Dinner:
m	Breakfast:	Lunch:	Dinner:
t	Breakfast:	Lunch:	Dinner:
w	Breakfast:	Lunch:	Dinner:
t	Breakfast:	Lunch:	Dinner:
f	Breakfast:	Lunch:	Dinner:
s	Breakfast:	Lunch:	Dinner:

Daily Food Tracker

BREAKFAST

Carb   :

Protein :

Fat   :

Sugar   :

Total Calorie :

LUNCH

Carb   :

Protein :

Fat   :

Sugar   :

Total Calorie :

DINNER

Carb   :

Protein :

Fat   :

Sugar   :

Total Calorie :

SNACK

Carb   :

Protein :

Fat   :

Sugar   :

Total Calorie :

WATER INTAKE

NOTE

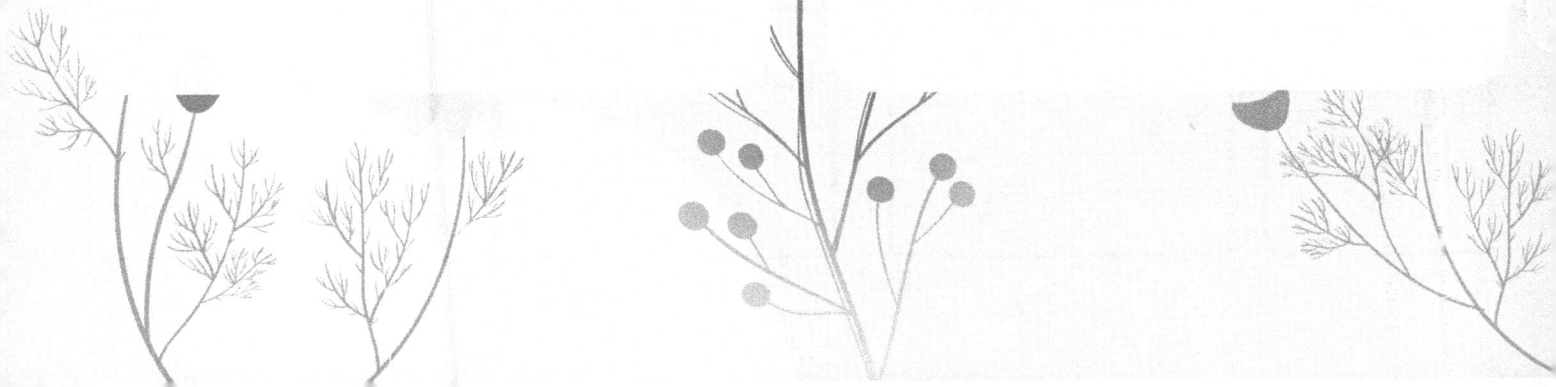

Before & After

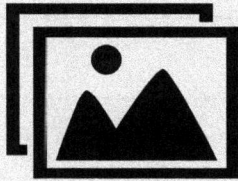

BEFORE PHOTO

STARTS

	WEIGHT	
	MUSCLE	
	BODY FAT	
	BMI	

MEASUREMENTS

	CHEST	
	BICEPS	
	HIPS	
	CALVES	
	WAIST	
	THIGHS	

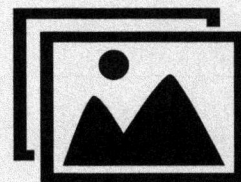

AFTER PHOTO

My Notes